PUBLISHED BY NICHOLAS THOMPSON

Soups: Eat All You Want and Still Lose Weight

@ Jamie Katz

Published By Nicholas Thompson

@ Jamie Katz

Soups: Eat All You Want and Still Lose Weight

All Right RESERVED

ISBN 978-87-975002-5-5

TABLE OF CONTENTS

chapter 1 1

   Understanding Nutrients And Its Importance To Your Body 1

Sprouts-Potato Soup 9

Mix-Veg Stock 11

Baby Corn – Vegetable Thick Soup 13

Low Fodmap Tortilla Soup 15

Creamy Mustard Soup 19

Low Fodmap Beef Ramen 21

Low Fodmap Goulash Soup 23

Healthy Green Food Juice 24

Pomegranate Juice Cranberry Juice 26

Gooseberry Orange Juice 27

Watermelon Strawberry Tomato Juice 28

How To Make Chicken Stew With Chickpeas And Plum Tomatoes 29

Italian Leek And Potato Soup 32

Lemony Chicken Soup (Chicken Avgolemono) 35

3. Doughnuts In Orange And Ginger Glaze 39

Easy Raw Breakfast Balls 41

Lemon Scones With Blackberry Sage 43

Oat Meal Raw Classic 45

Strawberry And Banana Crepes Raw Food Style 47

Lentil Soup With Tomatoes And Spinach 49

Tomato Soup 53

Lentil Detox Soup 55

Spinach Soup 57

Tomato Detox Soup 59

Green Soup 60

Broccoli Soup 62

Cabbage Fat-Burning Soup 64

Hot And Sour Chicken And Cabbage Soup 66

Thai Chicken Cabbage Soup 69

Cabbage Patch Soup 72

Cabbage, Potato And Baked Bean Soup 73

- Broccoli Cheddar Soup 75
- Yummy Tomato Soup 78
- Happy Wedding Soup 80
- Mia's Chicken Noodle Soup.. 82
- Cream Of Broccoli Soup 84
- Cream Of Potato Soup.. 86
- Cream Of Cauliflower Soup 88
- Broth Based Soup 90
- Corn Chips In Good Ol' Raw Guacamole 91
- Easy Raw Onion Rings 94
- Kale Chips 96
- Lemon-Coconut Squares 97
- Pepper Poppers, Pine Nut Filling And Eggplant Bacon... 98
- Crockpot Corn And Sausage Chowder 101
- Michael Romano's Secret-Ingredient Soup.................. 103
- Turkey And Italian Sausage Chili 106
- Double Lentil And Mushroom Barley Soup 109
- Creamy Vegan Tomato Soup.. 114

Masala Tomato Soup 117

Tomato Soup In Coconut Milk 120

Tomato-Onion Soup 123

Low Fodmap Tomato Soup With Meatballs 126

Low Fodmap Chicken Noodle Soup 130

Low Fodmap Pumpkin Noodle Soup 132

Spinach Cucumber Orange Juice 136

Spinach Black Carrots Beetroot Juice 137

Carrots Peas Ginger Grape Juice 138

Pineapple Ginger Lemon Juice 139

Chapter 1
Understanding Nutrients and its importance to your body

What is nutrition?

Nutrition is essential to sustain a healthy and normal life span. The need starts from the infant stage and goes on right till old age. Food is necessary for providing nutrition to the human body system. Nutrition has a direct connection between our health, diet, minor and major ailments and how we can prevent them from occurring. Through food we get nutrition in the form of nutrients.

What Are Nutrients?

Nutrients as the word goes have a direct connection with nutrition that is required by the human body. Nutrients help a life to grow, develop into a perfect being and blossom.

It may seem surprising to know that there are a multitude of nutrients available in the food stuffs available in the market that most of us are unaware of. Need of the hour is to become aware of them and alter our eating tastes and accept a healthier eating regimen. One should incorporate a well-balanced diet comprising of vegetables, leafy greens, fruits, whole grains, lean meats, dairy and poultry to obtain the required nutrients, vitamins and minerals needed to remain fit and fine.

Nutrients are basically food components that are made up of carbohydrates, proteins, fats, vitamins, minerals, amino acids and H_2O. These are indispensable for development and maintenance of life. Though there are innumerable nutrients, but still there are a few essential nutrients that should be added to your diet. Nutrients can be defined into two groups namely macro-nutrients and micro-nutrients.

Macro-nutrients

Macro-nutrients are of two types - one type provides energy while the other type doesn't but either way these nutrients are required in large quantities. Macro-nutrients provide carbs, protein and fat through which we get calories that are essential to energize the body to perform necessary bodily functions to stay healthy. Read on to know the role that carbs, protein and fats play in our existence on Planet Earth.

Carbohydrates

The basic function of carbs is to provide energy for the body. They provide calories that are needed by the body to perform day-to-day activities such as sitting, moving around, talking, driving, running, creative works, picking or moving objects and even sleeping. Calories also take care of the digestive system and are also take active part in the steady flow of blood in the body, maintaining the rhythmic beating of the heart as well as regulating body temperature and blood pressure. Foods such as potatoes, wheat, rice, beans, corns, sweet potatoes, yucca, fruits, bread provide substantial quantities of starch for generating carbs to provide energy to the body.

Proteins

Nutrients such as proteins can be termed as building blocks and sentinels that start being helpful right from pre-birth to adulthood. It helps in repairing injuries of the body, tissue change & growth and creates new blood in a duration of every few months. They provide amino acids to the body that help in the structure of bones & muscle growth and strengthen immune cells to combat infection, fight diseases and inflammation. Popular protein providing foods are legumes and soybeans, fish and seafood, mutton, beef, pork and poultry products such as eggs & chicken.

Fats

Fats are obtained from vegetable oils, milk, whey, cheese, coconut, nuts, fish and poultry and help in oiling the body cells and cushioning membranes for preventing damage to them. They are an integral part of the digestive system and help in absorbing fat-soluble vitamins obtained from food.

Fiber

We get fiber from carbohydrates. It is a basic part of food that we consume and assists in fuel for gut bacteria, health and nutrition. This is the part of food that the body doesn't absorb completely and neither does too much of starch and sugar finds its way into the blood stream. Fiber is essential for nutrition, health, and fuel for gut bacteria.

Water

Since the body is made up of more than 65% of water, it is very essential to keep the body hydrated with at least 3 to 6 liters of water per day to save it from dehydrating. Water is the rejuvenating factor that is closely associated with age, body mass, physical activities, dietary habits and gut health, to keep us healthy and on the move.

Micro-nutrients

Micro-nutrients as the name goes are required in little quantities. Micro-nutrients are made up of minerals, vitamins and phytochemicals that help the body to function to optimum capacity. Calories aren't obtained from them but still they are an indelible requirement of the body. Micro-nutrients comprise of minerals, vitamins and phytochemicals which play a crucial role in influencing general health and aid in neurological functions and cell metabolism.

Minerals such as potassium, chloride, sodium, magnesium and calcium are a necessity for the body and help in the formation of the skeletal structure as well as maintaining blood pressure and cardiovascular health. Iron helps the smooth passage of oxygen through the blood streams and prevents anemia.

Vitamins give us that spark of energy and assist in healing during injuries, immunity against diseases,

Vitamin A averts eye ailments & Vitamin E is good for skin health and bone formation.

Sprouts-Potato Soup

Ingredients:

- 2 tsp Corn Flour
- 2 tsp Butter
- ¼ tsp Black Pepper Powder
- Salt to taste
- 1 cup fresh Sprouts
- 1 medium sized Potato (boiled and then diced)
- 1 medium sized Onion (finely diced)
- 1 tbsp Celery (chopped)
- 1 tbsp Parsley (chopped)

Directions:

1. Steam-cook the sprouts and dice the boiled potato and then make a paste of sprouts and potato using a blender.
2. Take ½ a cup of fresh water and mix 2 tsp of corn flour in it and set it aside.
3. Heat the butter in a pan and then add diced onion, chopped celery and chopped parsley to the pan and stir for a minute.
4. Then add ½ cup of fresh water to the pan and cover it with a lid to let the veggies cook over a medium heat.
5. Remove the lid after 4-5 minutes and add the sprouts-potato paste to the vegetables followed by 1 cup of water and bring it to a boil.
6. Then add corn flour mixture to this boiling soup followed by salt and black pepper powder.
7. Keep stirring for 2-3 minutes more, garnish with grated coconut pulp and serve hot.

Mix-Veg Stock

Ingredients:

- 2 medium sized Onions
- 2 cups grated Cabbage
- ¼ tsp Garam Masala
- 1 cup diced Bottle Gourd
- 2 medium sized Potatoes
- Salt to taste

Directions:

1. Dice the bottle gourd, potatoes and onion.
2. Then mix all the vegetables together, add 6-7 cups of fresh water to them and steam-cook them.
3. Once cooked, blend all of the vegetables together using a blender.

4. Add salt and garam masala to this stock.
5. This stock can be mixed with salads and used as filler while making thick soups.

Baby Corn – Vegetable Thick Soup

Ingredients:

- 2 tsp Butter
- ¼ tsp Black Pepper Powder
- ¼ tsp Nutmeg Powder
- 2 cups White Stock
- 1 tbsp Celery (finely chopped)
- 1 ½ tsp grated Indian Cottage Cheese (*Paneer*)
- 1 ½ cup boiled Baby Corns (finely diced)
- 1 cup Spring Onions (finely diced)
- 2 tsp Wheat Flour
- 1/2 cup Milk
- Salt to taste

Directions:

1. Heat the butter in a pan and then add diced spring onions and chopped celery to the pan and stir till the onions are cooked.
2. Then add the wheat flour to the pan and stir for a minute and turn off the heat.
3. Now slowly add the white stock and milk to the contents of the pan and mix them thoroughly.
4. Turn on the heat again and add boiled baby corns, salt, black pepper powder and Nutmeg powder to the pan and let it cook for around 6-7 minutes.
5. (Add ½ a cup of water while cooking if needed to adjust the thickness)
6. Bring the soup to a boil and then garnish with chopped coriander leaves and grated cottage cheese. Serve hot.

low fodmap tortilla soup

INGREDIENTS:

- 1 tsp turmeric
- 1 tsp oregano
- 1/2 tsp chilli
- 1/4 tsp cayenne pepper
- 1/4 tsp cinnamon
- Pepper and salt
- 500 ml vegetable broth (make sure the broth is low FODMAP)
- 200 g canned diced tomatoes*
- 1 large carrot
- 1 bell pepper*
- 1 tsp cumin
- 1 tsp paprika

FOR THE TOPPING

- Lactose-free cream cheese or sour cream (sour cream only if you tolerate lactose)
- Grated cheese
- Black olives, in pieces
- 30 g sweet corn
- Spring onions, the green part
- 4 corn tortillas

DIRECTIONS:

1. Cut the bell pepper and the carrot into pieces.
2. Heat some oil in a pan. Add the bell pepper and carrot and fry for a few minutes until softened.
3. Add the vegetable broth, the tomato cubes and add all the spices.
4. Bring the soup to a boil. Then lower the heat and leave it to simmer for about 15-20 minutes.
5. Use an immersion blender to turn the soup into a smooth mixture. Blend only shortly if you like to have some pieces in your soup.
6. Taste the soup and add some extra spices if necessary.
7. While the soup simmers, heat the oven to 180 degrees Celcius (350 degrees Fahrenheit).
8. Cut the corn tortillas into strips. Put them on a baking sheet covered with baking parchment and sprinkle with a bit of oil and sea salt. Bake

the corn tortillas in the oven for about 15 minutes.
9. Divide the soup over two bowls. Top with the corn, olives, spring onion and cream cheese and sprinkle grated cheese on top. Serve with the homemade tortilla chips.

creamy mustard soup

INGREDIENTS:

- 200 ml rice cream (I use the rice cream from Alpro Soya)
- 100 g bacon (check the ingredients to make sure they are low FODMAP)
- 2–3 tbsp mustard
- 50 g butter (if you want to make this recipe entirely lactose-free you can use margarine)
- 60 g gluten-free flour
- 1.25 – 1.5 litre stock
- Pepper and salt

DIRECTIONS:

1. Melt the butter in a pan. Add the flour and stir through with a spoon. Like this you make roux. Stir the roux and leave it to cook on low

heat for about 3 minutes. Continue to stir now and then to keep it from burning.
2. Pour the stock into the pan carefully. Start with 1.25 litre. If you notice later on that the soup is too thick, you can add some extra stock.
3. Stir the soup with a whisk to remove any lumps. Lower the heat and leave the soup to boil for about 10 minutes.
4. In the meantime, fry the bacon until crisp.
5. Add the mustard to the soup. Taste the soup and add some more mustard and pepper and salt if necessary. Finally add the rice cream and heat through.
6. Serve the soup with the bacon

low fodmap beef ramen

INGREDIENTS:

- 1 tbsp tamarind paste or 2 tbsp soy sauce

- spring onion, only the green part

- fresh cilantro

- 1/2 tsp ground cumin

- 1 tsp smoked paprika

- 1/2 tsp cayenne pepper

- 3 blocks spelt ramen (about 180 g), gluten-free soba noodles or rice noodles*

- 300 g (0.6 pounds) beef, in cubes

- 150 g (1 cup) carrot

- 1.5 liter (6 cups) stock (I used three stock cubes to make this, check the ingredients on the package to make sure you use low FODMAP stock cubes)

- pepper and salt

DIRECTIONS:

1. Heat 1.5 liter of stock in a pan. Add the cubed beef and leave to simmer on low heat for 1 to 1.5 hours, until the beef is fully cooked and tender.
2. Cut the carrot into small pieces. Add them to the soup. Add some rings of spring onion and the tamarind paste too.
3. Season the soup with cumin, paprika, cayenne pepper, pepper and salt and leave the soup to simmer for another 15 minutes.
4. Finally add the noodles and leave them to simmer for 10 minutes until they have softened. Taste the soup and add some extra spices if necessary.
5. Divide the soup over the bowls and serve with some extra spring onion and fresh cilantro.

low fodmap goulash soup

INGREDIENTS:

- 1 tbsp tomato paste
- ½ tsp ground paprika
- ¼ tsp ground cumin
- 200 ml red wine
- 1 liter stock (make sure to use low FODMAP stock cubes)
- 100 g green beans, in pieces
- 75 g bacon strips
- 400 g beef stew meat
- 2 tbsp olive oil
- green bell pepper*
- Pepper and salt

- Optional: 2 tbsp lactose-free cream cheese or sour cream

DIRECTIONS:

1. Cut the meat and the paprika into cubes.
2. Bake the bacon for a few minutes in a soup pan. Add the paprika, tomato paste, ground paprika, ground cumin and bake for two minutes.
3. Add the stock and the red wine. Stir together and bring the soup to a boil. Cover and leave the soup to simmer for 2 hours.
4. Add the green beans to the soup and boil for another 20 minutes. Season the soup with pepper and salt.
5. Serve the goulash soup with a scoop of lactose-free cream cheese or sour cream.

Healthy green food juice

Ingredients:

- 4 leaves of kale
- 4 oranges peeled and seeds removed
- 1 green apple
- 1 cup of grapes
- 2 bunches of fresh spinach
- 1 cabbage
- Juice of 1 lemon

DIRECTIONS:

1. Add the fruits and vegetables in the blender except for the lemon and mix well.
2. Pour it into glasses filled with ice cubes.
3. Squeeze lemon juice.

Pomegranate juice Cranberry juice

Ingredients:

- 2 beets peeled and diced
- 2 cups of ripe red cranberries
- Juice of 1 lemon
- 2 large pomegranates peeled
- Powdered sugar for layering on glasses

DIRECTIONS:

1. Add the fruits and vegetables to the blender and mix well.
2. Squeeze the lemon into a small plate.
3. Dip the glasses in the lemon and dip them in the icing sugar.
4. Fill the glasses with ice cubes and pour in juice.

Gooseberry orange juice

Ingredients:

- 2 tbsp honey
- 1/2 cup of water
- 1/2 teaspoon of black salt
- 6 gooseberries seeded and cut into pieces
- 4 oranges peeled and seeds removed
- Ice cubes

DIRECTIONS:

1. Add oranges, gooseberries and water to the blender.
2. Add honey and black salt.
3. Mix it well with ice cubes to get a smooth consistency.
4. Pour on glasses.
5. This juice aids in weight loss.

Watermelon Strawberry Tomato juice

Ingredients:

- 2 large tomatoes
- 1/2 teaspoon of black salt
- Cut 6 watermelon cubes and remove seeds
- 10 pieces of strawberries
- Ice cubes

DIRECTIONS:

1. Add tomatoes and fruits to the blender.
2. Add ice cubes and mix well.
3. Layer it with black salt if served in glasses.

How to Make Chicken Stew with Chickpeas and Plum Tomatoes

Ingredients:

- 1 teaspoon ground cumin
- 1 teaspoon ground coriander
- 1 can (15 oz) chickpeas, drained and rinsed
- 1 can (14 oz) diced plum tomatoes
- 1 cup chicken broth
- 1/2 cup fresh parsley, chopped
- 4 boneless, skinless chicken breasts, cut into chunks
- 1 tablespoon olive oil
- 1 large onion, chopped
- 3 cloves garlic, minced
- Salt and freshly ground black pepper to taste

Directions:

1. Heat olive oil in a large, heavy-bottomed pot or Dutch oven over medium-high heat.
2. Add the chicken chunks and cook until they develop a golden-brown crust. Remove the chicken from the pot and set it aside.
3. In the same pot, add the chopped onion and sauté until it becomes translucent.
4. Add the minced garlic and sauté for an additional 30 seconds until fragrant.
5. Sprinkle the ground cumin and coriander over the onion and garlic. Stir to coat the aromatics with the spices.
6. Add the drained and rinsed chickpeas to the pot, stirring to combine.
7. Pour in the diced plum tomatoes, including their juice, and the chicken broth.
8. Return the seared chicken to the pot.
9. Bring the stew to a gentle boil, then reduce the heat to low, cover the pot, and let it

simmer for about 20-25 minutes. This allows the chicken to cook through and the flavors to meld.
10. Season the stew with salt and freshly ground black pepper to taste.
11. Stir in chopped fresh parsley just before serving to add a burst of fresh flavor.
12. Ladle the Chicken Stew with Chickpeas and Plum Tomatoes into bowls and enjoy it hot. It's delicious on its own or served with crusty bread, rice, or couscous.
13. This Chicken Stew with Chickpeas and Plum Tomatoes is a comforting and wholesome meal that embodies the Mediterranean and Middle Eastern culinary traditions. It's a flavorful combination of Ingredients: that results in a satisfying and nutritious dish. Enjoy it as a hearty dinner option on any occasion.

Italian Leek and Potato Soup

Ingredients:

- 2 cloves garlic, minced
- 4 cups (960ml) chicken or vegetable broth
- 2 tablespoons olive oil
- Salt and freshly ground black pepper to taste
- 3 leeks, white and light green parts only, cleaned and sliced
- 2 large potatoes, peeled and diced
- 1 onion, chopped
- Fresh parsley or chives for garnish (optional)

Directions:

1. Prepare the Leeks: Clean the leeks thoroughly, as they can trap dirt between their layers. Slice them into thin rounds, using only the white and light green parts.

2. Sauté the Aromatics: In a large pot, heat the olive oil over medium heat. Add the chopped onion and garlic and sauté for a few minutes until they become translucent.
3. Add Leeks and Potatoes: Add the sliced leeks and diced potatoes to the pot. Sauté them for a few more minutes, stirring occasionally.
4. Pour in the Broth: Pour in the chicken or vegetable broth, ensuring that the leeks and potatoes are covered. Season with a pinch of salt and freshly ground black pepper.
5. Simmer: Bring the mixture to a boil, then reduce the heat to low, cover the pot, and let the soup simmer for about 20-25 minutes, or until the potatoes become tender.
6. Blend the Soup: Once the potatoes are soft, use an immersion blender or a regular blender (in batches) to purée the soup until it reaches

your desired level of creaminess. Be careful when blending hot liquids.

7. Adjust Seasoning: Taste the soup and adjust the seasoning with more salt and pepper if needed.
8. Serve: Ladle the Italian Leek and Potato Soup into bowls. You can garnish it with chopped fresh parsley or chives if desired.
9. This soup is best enjoyed warm and is a comforting and nutritious option for any time of the year. It represents the Italian approach to combining simple Ingredients: to create dishes that are both delicious and healthful. Serve it with a slice of crusty bread for a satisfying meal.

Lemony Chicken Soup (Chicken Avgolemono)

Ingredients:

- Salt and freshly ground black pepper to taste
- 1 cup long-grain rice
- 4 large eggs
- Juice of 3-4 lemons
- 1 whole chicken (about 3-4 pounds) or bone-in chicken pieces
- 8 cups water
- 1 onion, chopped
- 2 carrots, chopped
- 2 celery stalks, chopped
- Fresh parsley, chopped, for garnish

Directions:

1. In a large pot, combine the chicken, water, chopped onion, carrots, and celery.
2. Bring the mixture to a boil, then reduce the heat to a simmer.
3. Skim off any foam that rises to the surface.
4. Cover and simmer for about 1.5 to 2 hours, or until the chicken is tender and fully cooked.
5. Once the chicken is cooked, remove it from the pot and set it aside to cool. When it's cool enough to handle, shred the chicken into bite-sized pieces. Discard the bones and skin.
6. Cook the Rice: In the same pot with the chicken broth, add the long-grain rice. Simmer for about 15-20 minutes, or until the rice is cooked and tender. Season with salt and pepper to taste.
7. Whisk the Eggs and Lemon Juice: In a separate bowl, whisk together the eggs and lemon juice until well combined.

8. Temper the Egg Mixture: Take a ladle of the hot chicken broth and slowly whisk it into the egg and lemon mixture. This step helps to temper the eggs, preventing them from curdling when added to the hot soup.
9. Add the Avgolemono to the Soup: Gradually pour the tempered egg mixture back into the pot of soup while stirring constantly. Keep the heat low to avoid curdling. Continue stirring until the soup thickens slightly.
10. Add the Shredded Chicken: Return the shredded chicken to the pot and stir to combine.
11. Taste and Adjust: Taste the soup and adjust the seasoning by adding more salt, pepper, or lemon juice if needed.
12. Serve: Ladle the Lemony Chicken Soup into bowls, garnish with chopped fresh parsley, and serve hot.

13. This comforting and nourishing Lemony Chicken Soup, or Avgolemono, combines the goodness of chicken, eggs, lemon, and rice to create a velvety and satisfying dish. It's a taste of Greek tradition that provides warmth and comfort, perfect for a cozy meal or when you need a bowl of flavorful soup to brighten your day. Enjoy the creamy, tangy delight of this timeless dish.

3. Doughnuts in Orange and Ginger Glaze

Ingredients:

For the Doughnuts:

- 1/3 cup raw and organic agave nectar
- 1/3 cup coconut oil, melted
- 1/4 cup coconut sugar
- 1 tsp. cinnamon
- 2 1/2 cups raw oat flour
- 1 cup Brazil nuts, finely grounded
- 1/4 cup raw and organic coconut flour
- 1 tsp. vanilla

For the Orange and Ginger Glaze:

- Zest from one orange
- 3 tbsp. orange juice
- 3 tbsp. raw coconut butter, softened

- 2 tbsp. raw and organic agave nectar
- 1 tsp. ginger, freshly grated

Directions:

For the Doughnuts:

1. Put all the Ingredients: in a large bowl, making sure that everything is well combined.
2. Make one doughnut at a time. Simply press firmly into the doughnut pan and then tip the pan over. Tap the pan to release the doughnut.
3. Pour the orange glaze on top of the doughnuts.

For the Orange Glaze:

4. Put all the Ingredients: in a bowl and whisk thoroughly.
5. Pour the glaze over the doughnuts.

Easy Raw Breakfast Balls

Ingredients:

- 1/4 cup yacon syrup
- 1/4 cup date paste
- 1/4 cup raisins, chopped
- 1/4 cup cranberries, chopped
- 2 tbsp. coconut oil, melted
- 2 tbsp. chia seeds
- 2 tbsp. hemp seeds
- 1/2 tsp. cinnamon
- Juice of half an orange
- Zest of 1 orange
- 1 cup raw almond flour
- 1/2 cup medjool dates, chopped
- 1/2 cup almonds, chopped

- 1/2 cup coconut, shredded
- 1/2 cup desiccated coconut
- Pinch of Himalayan sea salt

Directions:

1. Whisk the chia with the orange juice and the orange zest. Set the mixture aside.
2. In a separate bowl, mix all the other Ingredients: thoroughly.
3. Gradually combine the two mixtures together. Work the mixture with your hands while combining the two mixtures.
4. Using your hand, roll the mixture into ball shapes. Then roll the balls in the desiccated coconut.
5. Put the balls in the fridge and let it set before eating. If you want a crispier finish, you can then dehydrate the balls for 8 hours at 105F/40C.

Lemon Scones with Blackberry Sage

Ingredients:

For the Lemon Scones:

- 1/2 cup macadamia nuts, finely ground
- 1/2 cup coconut crystals
- 1/3 cup chia seeds
- 2 1/2 cups raw flaked oats, finely grounded into oat flour
- 1 cup almond milk
- 2 lemons, zest and juice

For the Blackberry Sage:

- 1 1/2 tbsp. chia seeds
- 1 1/2 tbsp. dried sage
- 1 cup blackberries
- 2 tbsp. agave nectar

Directions:

For the Lemon Scones:

1. In a large bowl, combine the oat flour with the chia seeds, ground macadamia nuts and the coconut crystals.
2. Add in the lemon juice, zest and the almond milk. Let the mixture rest for about 5 minutes.
3. Get the mixture and form it into 1-inch thick circle. Put it on a non-stick and cut into 8 wedges.
4. Dehydrate this for about 45 minutes at 145F/63C. Then reduce the heat to 115F/46C and continue dehydrating for about 7 hours.

For the Blackberry Sage:

5. Put all Ingredients: in a food processor and puree.
6. Place the mixture in a bowl and refrigerate for about 30 minutes.

Oat Meal Raw Classic

Ingredients:

- 1 banana
- 1 tbsp. golden flax seed, soaked overnight
- 2 tsp. cinnamon
- 2 apples
- Purified water

Directions:

1. Soak the flax seeds in purified water overnight.
2. Peel the apples and cut into smaller parts. Peel the banana and cut into parts. Rinse the flax seeds.
3. Place all the Ingredients: in the blender and put on high speed. Add about 1/4 cup of water to let the mixture really blend well.

Continue blending until the mixture is smooth.

Strawberry and Banana Crepes Raw Food Style

Ingredients:

For the Crepes:

- 4 bananas
- Juice of 1 lemon

For the Cashew Vanilla Cream:

- 1 cup cashews, soaked overnight
- Pulp from 2 young coconuts
- Splash of Madagascar vanilla

Directions:

For the Crepes:

1. Put the bananas in a food processor along with the lemon juice. Process until the mixture turns to liquid.
2. Place the mixture into 5-inch round pans and spread the mixture evenly.

3. Dehydrate the mixture overnight at 115F/46C.

For the Cashew Vanilla Cream:

1. Put the cashews in a blender and blend on high speed.
2. Add the coconut meat and the vanilla into the blender, making sure that everything is well combined.
3. Refrigerate the mixture to thicken.

Lentil Soup with Tomatoes and Spinach

Ingredients:

- 1 celery stalk, diced
- 1 can (14.5 oz) diced tomatoes
- 6 cups vegetable or chicken broth
- 1 teaspoon ground cumin
- 1 teaspoon ground coriander
- 1/2 teaspoon ground paprika
- Salt and freshly ground black pepper to taste
- 3 cups fresh spinach, chopped
- 1 cup dried green or brown lentils, rinsed and drained
- 1 tablespoon olive oil
- 1 onion, chopped
- 2 cloves garlic, minced

- 1 carrot, diced
- Juice of 1 lemon
- Fresh parsley or cilantro for garnish (optional)

Directions:

1. Rinse the lentils thoroughly in a fine-mesh strainer, and set them aside to drain.

2. In a large soup pot or Dutch oven, heat the olive oil over medium heat. Add the chopped onion and cook until it becomes translucent, about 5 minutes.
3. Add the minced garlic, diced carrot, and diced celery. Sauté for an additional 3-4 minutes until the vegetables start to soften.
4. Stir in the rinsed lentils, diced tomatoes (including their juice), ground cumin, ground coriander, ground paprika, salt, and freshly

ground black pepper. Cook for 2-3 minutes, allowing the flavors to meld.
5. Add the vegetable or chicken broth to the pot and bring the mixture to a boil. Reduce the heat to a simmer, cover the pot, and let it cook for about 20-25 minutes, or until the lentils are tender but not mushy.
6. Stir in the chopped fresh spinach and continue to simmer for an additional 3-5 minutes until the spinach wilts and becomes tender.
7. Squeeze the juice of one lemon into the soup and stir to combine. The lemon juice adds a zesty, bright flavor.
8. Taste the soup and adjust the seasoning with more salt and pepper if needed.
9. Ladle the Lentil Soup with Tomatoes and Spinach into bowls. Garnish with fresh parsley or cilantro if desired. Serve hot.
10. This hearty and nutritious Lentil Soup with Tomatoes and Spinach is a comforting choice

for a healthy and satisfying meal. It's perfect for lunch or dinner and pairs well with crusty bread or a simple side salad. Enjoy the fusion of flavors and the nutritional benefits of this dish.

Tomato Soup

Ingredients:

- 2 cloves garlic, minced
- 1 stalk celery, diced
- 1 carrot, diced
- 2 tablespoons extra virgin olive oil, divided
- 2 cups low sodium vegetable broth
- ½ teaspoon sea salt
- 1 bay leaf
- Dash of cayenne pepper
- ¼ cup chopped fresh basil
- 2 medium shallots, chopped
- 1 pound fresh tomatoes, sliced in half

Directions:

1. Preheat the oven to 400 degrees F.

2. Place the sliced tomatoes on a cookie sheet lined with foil. Drizzle 1 tablespoon of oil over tomatoes and roast them for 20 minutes.
3. In a small skillet, sauté diced carrot and celery in the remaining 1 tablespoon of oil over medium-low heat until tender. Add garlic and shallots then turn the heat to low and continue to sauté for another 4 minutes.
4. Remove the tomatoes from the oven and allow cool before peeling them. Discard the peelings.
5. Add all the Ingredients: into a food processor, apart from the broth and process until smooth.
6. Add the tomato puree mixture and broth to a medium pot, bring to a boil, lower the heat and simmer for 15-20 minutes. Remove bay leaf and serve.

Lentil Detox Soup

Ingredients:

- 1 teaspoon cumin powder
- 1 teaspoon turmeric powder
- 3 garlic cloves, crushed
- 1 onion, peeled and cut in quarters
- 1 parsnip, peeled and roughly chopped
- 3 carrots, peeled and roughly chopped
- 1 sweet potato, peeled and cut into cubes
- Fresh parsley, for garnish
- ½ cup cooked red lentils
- 1 teaspoon coconut oil
- ½ inch piece of ginger, peeled and grated
- 2 cups low sodium vegetable broth, warm
- ¼ teaspoon sea salt

- Pinch of chili powder
- 1 teaspoon coconut milk for garnish

Directions:

1. Preheat the oven to 329 degrees F.
2. Use a baking paper to line a baking sheet then garlic, onion, parsnip, carrots, and sweet potato and then season with chili, turmeric, cumin and salt. Add coconut oil and toss to combine.
3. Roast for 20 minutes then transfer to a blender.
4. Add the warm vegetable broth, cooked red lentils and grated ginger into the blender and process until smooth.
5. Garnish with fresh parsley and coconut milk, and serve warm.

Spinach Soup

Ingredients:

- Ground black pepper to taste
- ¼ teaspoon salt
- 1 clove garlic, minced
- 1 medium onion, coarsely chopped
- 1 tablespoon rosemary, finely chopped
- 6 cups spinach leaves
- 4 cup chicken or vegetable broth or water
- 2 cups red potatoes, peeled and diced
- 2 tablespoons extra-virgin olive oil

Directions:

1. Preheat the oven to 375 degrees F
2. Add olive oil into a large saucepan over medium heat. Once hot, add garlic, onions,

rosemary, salt, and pepper. Reduce heat to medium-low and cook, as you stir occasionally for 5 minutes
3. Put in the potatoes and cook, occasionally stirring for 3 minutes.
4. Pour in the broth or water and simmer over medium heat.
5. Cook the potatoes until they are soft then stir in the spinach. Simmer the greens until they are tender.
6. Puree the soup using an immersion blender, leaving it a little chunky as desired.
7. Serve the soup and enjoy.

Tomato Detox Soup

Ingredients:

- 4-6 whole dried chipotle chiles
- 1 teaspoon dried oregano flakes
- 2 large carrots, sliced into half-moons
- 2 cloves garlic, finely chopped
- ½ bunch Swiss chard, stems separated from leaves both chopped
- 1 yellow onion, diced
- 2 large stalks celery, sliced
- 1 teaspoon sea salt
- 1 cup frozen fire-roasted corn
- 6 cups low-sodium vegetables broth
- 1 teaspoon ground cumin

- 1 15-oz. jar diced unsalted tomatoes with juices
- 2 tablespoons extra-virgin olive oil

Directions:

1. Heat olive oil in a large pot over medium heat. Add onions, celery, carrots, garlic and chard stems; sauté until tender.
2. Add chiles, oregano, cumin, tomatoes, and sauté for 2 minutes. Stir in salt, broth, and corn. Bring the mixture to a boil then cover and reduce the heat to a simmer and cook until carrots are tender.
3. Stir in the chard leaves and turn off the heat.
4. Serve and enjoy.

Green Soup

Ingredients:

- 6 kale leaves

- 1 small head of broccoli
- 2 cloves garlic
- 1 leek
- 4 cups vegetable stock
- 2 sticks celery
- 1-2 zucchini
- A handful of parsley

Directions:

1. Wash and chop all veggies.
2. Heat the oil lightly in a pot over low heat. Add garlic and leeks and continue cooking on low heat.
3. Add the vegetables and vegetable stock then slowly bring to a boil and cook until the zucchini is soft.
4. Add the salt and pepper to taste
5. Process the soup using an immersion blender leaving it as chunky as you prefer.

Broccoli Soup

Ingredients:

- 1 carrot, peeled and finely chopped
- 1 parsnip, peeled and finely chopped
- 1 cup greens
- 2 cloves garlic, crushed
- 1 onion, finely diced
- 2 celery stalks, finely diced
- 2 cups broccoli florets
- Toasted mixed seeds and nuts
- 1 tablespoon chia seeds
- 1 teaspoon coconut oil
- Juice from ½ lemon
- ½ teaspoon salt

- 2 cups filtered water
- 1 teaspoon coconut milk

Directions:

1. Heat coconut oil in a soup pot. Add the onion, garlic, parsnip, carrot, celery stick, and broccoli. Cook over low heat for 5 minutes stirring frequently.
2. Add the filtered water and bring to a boil, then cover the pot with lid and let it simmer for 5-7 minutes, until the vegetables are tender but mushy.
3. Stir in greens, and then transfer to a blender. Add the chia seeds and lemon juice and process until smooth.
4. Serve and top with toasted seeds and nuts.

Cabbage Fat-Burning Soup

INGREDIENTS:

- 1 (15 ounce) can cut green beans, drained
- 2 quarts tomato juice
- 2 green bell peppers, diced
- 10 stalks celery, chopped
- 1 (14 ounce) can beef broth
- 5 carrots, chopped
- 3 onions, chopped
- 2 (16 ounce) cans whole peeled tomatoes, with liquid
- 1 large head cabbage, chopped
- 1 (1 ounce) envelope dry onion soup mix

Directions:

1. Place carrots, onions, tomatoes, cabbage, green beans, peppers, and celery in a large pot.
2. Add onion soup mix, tomato juice, beef broth, and enough water to cover vegetables.
3. Simmer until vegetables are tender. May be stored in the refrigerator for several days.

Hot and Sour Chicken and Cabbage Soup

Ingredients:

- 1 tablespoon black pepper
- 1 teaspoon garlic powder
- 1 onion, cut in strips
- 1 teaspoon olive oil
- ½ pound skinless, boneless chicken breast meat - cubed
- ½ head cabbage, shredded
- 1 cup fresh bean sprouts
- 2 eggs, beaten
- 10 cups chicken broth
- 1 teaspoon hot pepper flakes
- ¼ cup red wine vinegar
- ¼ cup soy sauce

- 1 tablespoon minced lemon grass
- 1 tablespoon fish sauce
- ¼ cup chopped fresh parsley

Directions:

1. Pour chicken broth into a large pot. Stir in hot pepper flakes, vinegar, soy sauce, lemon grass, fish sauce, black pepper, garlic powder, and onion. Bring to a boil over high heat, then lessen warmness to medium-low and keep at a simmer.
2. Meanwhile, heat olive oil in a skillet over medium-high heat. Stir in cubed chicken, and prepare dinner dinner until no longer pink in the center, approximately five minutes.
3. Stir chicken into the simmering soup along with the cabbage and bean sprouts. Simmer until the cabbage is tender, about 10 minutes.
4. Remove the pot from the warmness, and slowly stir in the beaten egg, then gently stir

withinside the chopped parsley. Serve immediately.

Thai Chicken Cabbage Soup

Ingredients:

- 6 carrots, cut into 1 inch pieces
- 1 medium head cabbage, shredded
- 1 (8 ounce) package uncooked egg noodles
- 1 teaspoon Thai chile sauce
- 3 skinless, boneless chicken breast halves
- 8 cups chicken broth
- 2 leeks, sliced

Directions:

1. Pour chicken broth into a large pot. Stir in hot pepper flakes, vinegar, soy sauce, lemon grass, fish sauce, black pepper, garlic powder, and onion. Bring to a boil over high heat, then lessen warmth to medium-low and keep at a simmer.

2. Meanwhile, heat olive oil in a skillet over medium-high heat. Stir in cubed chicken, and prepare dinner dinner until no longer pink in the center, approximately five minutes. Stir chicken into the simmering soup along with the cabbage and bean sprouts. Simmer until the cabbage is tender, about 10 minutes.
3. Remove the pot from the warmth, and slowly stir in the beaten egg, then gently stir withinside the chopped parsley. Serve immediately.
4. Place chicken breasts and broth in to a stockpot or Dutch oven. Bring to a boil and let simmer for about 20 minutes, or till chicken is cooked through. Remove the chicken from the broth and set aside to cool.
5. Put the leeks and carrots into the pot and simmer them for 10 minutes, or until tender. Shred the cooled chook in to bite sized portions and return it to the pot. Add the

cabbage and egg noodles and cook another five minutes or until the noodles are soft. The soup has to be thick like a stew. Serve warm and flavor to taste with Thai chili sauce.

Cabbage Patch Soup

Ingredients:

- 2 cups shredded cabbage
- 1 cup sliced carrots
- 1 teaspoon salt
- ¼ teaspoon ground black pepper
- 1 bay leaves
- 1 cup frozen green peas
- 1 tablespoon olive oil
- 3 tablespoons bacon bits
- 1 onion, chopped
- 1 tablespoon all-purpose flour
- 3 (14.5 ounce) cans chicken broth
- ¾ cup sour cream

Directions:

1. Heat the oil in a large saucepan over medium heat. Saute the bacon bits and onion in the oil for about five minutes, or until onion is tender.
2. Stir in the flour to coat well, then quickly pour in the chicken broth. Stir continuously for three minutes, or until particularly thickened.
3. Next, add the cabbage, carrots, salt, ground black pepper and bay leaf. Reduce heat to low and simmer for 20 minutes.
4. Stir in the peas and sour cream 1 minute earlier than serving. Allow to heat thru and remove bay leaf.

Cabbage, Potato and Baked Bean Soup

Ingredients:

- 6 cups shredded cabbage
- 4 cups chicken broth
- 1 bay leaf

- ½ teaspoon ground black pepper
- 2 teaspoons vegetable oil
- 2½ cups peeled and cubed potatoes
- 1 cup thinly sliced celery
- 1 onion, chopped
- 1 (15 ounce) can pork and beans in tomato sauce

Directions:

1. Heat oil in medium size saucepan. Add potatoes, celery, and onion, saute for 5 minutes.
2. Stir in cabbage, cover and cook over medium heat, until cabbage is tender.
3. Add broth, bay leaf, pepper and pork and beans. Heat until soup is hot and then remove bay leaf and serve.

Broccoli Cheddar Soup

Ingredients:

- 2 cups chicken stock
- 1 1/2 cups coarsely chopped broccoli florets
- 1 cup carrots (matchstick cut)
- 1 stalk celery (thinly sliced)
- 2 1/2 cups shredded sharp Cheddar cheese
- 1 tablespoon butter
- 1/2 onion (chopped)
- 1/4 cup melted butter
- 1/4 cup flour
- 2 cups milk
- salt and ground black pepper

Directions:

1. Melt 1 tablespoon butter in a skillet over medium-high heat. Saute onion in hot butter until translucent, about 5 minutes. Set aside.
2. Whisk 1/4 cup melted butter and flour together in a large saucepan over medium-low heat; cook until flour loses it's granular texture, adding 1 to 2 tablespoons of milk if necessary to keep the flour from burning, 3 to 4 minutes.
3. Gradually pour milk into flour mixture while whisking constantly. Stir chicken stock into milk mixture.
4. Bring to a simmer; cook until flour taste is gone and mixture is thickened, about 20 minutes.
5. Add broccoli, carrots, sauteed onion, and celery; simmer until vegetables are tender, about 20 minutes.

6. Stir Cheddar cheese into vegetable mixture until cheese melts. Season with salt and pepper to taste.

Yummy Tomato Soup

Ingredients:

- 2 cups chicken broth
- 2 tablespoons butter
- 2 tablespoons all-purpose flour
- 1 teaspoon salt
- 4 cups chopped fresh tomatoes
- 1 slice onion
- 4 whole cloves
- 2 teaspoons white sugar

Directions:

1. In a stockpot, over medium heat, combine the tomatoes, onion, cloves and chicken broth.
2. Bring to a boil, and gently boil for about 20 minutes to blend all of the flavors.

3. Remove from heat and run the mixture through a food mill into a large bowl. Discard any stuff left over in the food mill.
4. In the now empty stockpot, melt the butter over medium heat. Stir in the flour to make a roux, cooking until the roux is a medium brown.
5. Gradually whisk in a bit of the tomato mixture, so that no lumps form, then stir in the rest. Season with sugar and salt, and adjust to taste.

Happy Wedding Soup

Ingredients:

- 1 tablespoon grated Parmesan cheese
- 1/2 teaspoon dried basil
- 1/2 teaspoon onion powder
- 5 3/4 cups chicken broth
- 2 cups thinly sliced escarole
- 1 cup uncooked orzo pasta
- 1/2 pound extra-lean ground beef
- 1 egg(beaten)
- 2 tablespoons dry bread crumbs
- 1/3 cup finely chopped carrot

Directions:

1. In medium bowl, combine meat, egg, bread crumbs, cheese, basil and onion powder; shape into 3/4 inch balls.
2. In large saucepan, heat broth to boiling; stir in escarole, orzo pasta, chopped carrot and meatballs.
3. Return to boil, then reduce heat to medium. Cook at slow boil for 10 minutes, Stir frequently to prevent sticking.

Mia's Chicken Noodle Soup

Ingredients:

- 1 1/2 tablespoons salt
- 1 teaspoon poultry seasoning
- 1 cup chopped celery
- 1 cup chopped onion
- 1/3 cup cornstarch
- 1/4 cup water
- 2 1/2 cups wide egg noodles
- 1 teaspoon vegetable oil
- 12 cups chicken broth
- 3 cups chicken meat(diced & cooked)

Directions:

1. Bring a large pot of lightly salted water to a boil. Add egg noodles and oil, and boil for 8

minutes, or until tender. Drain, and rinse under cool running water.
2. In a large saucepan or Dutch oven, combine broth, salt, and poultry seasoning. Bring to a boil.
3. Stir in celery and onion. Reduce heat, cover, and simmer 15 minutes.
4. In a small bowl, mix cornstarch and water together until cornstarch is completely dissolved.
5. Gradually add to soup, stirring constantly. Stir in noodles and chicken, and heat through.

CREAM OF BROCCOLI SOUP

Ingredients:

- 4 Cups chicken broth
- 2 potatoes, cubed
- 2 Cups milk
- 1 Cup cheddar cheese, shredded
- salt and pepper to taste
- 1 Tablespoon olive oil
- 1 onion, grated
- 1-2 bunches of fresh broccoli cut or one bag frozen broccoli

DIRECTIONS:

1. Heat oil in soup pan and cook onion and potato cubes. Saute. Season with salt and pepper. Add chicken broth and cook until potatoes are slightly tender.

2. Add broccoli to soup pan. Cook until broccoli and potatoes are tender. Add milk and cheese and stir until cheese is melted.
3. Add to blender and puree into cream soup or use an immersion blender.

CREAM OF POTATO SOUP

INGREDIENTS:

- 1 celery stalk
- 1 cup cauliflower pieces
- Water to cover
- 2 teaspoons chicken bouillon or 2 cubes
- 1/4 Cup milk
- 2 Cups potatoes, cubed
- 1 small onion, optional
- 1 carrot

DIRECTIONS:

1. Cut vegetables into slices or cubes. In soup pan place potatoes, onion, carrot, celery and cauliflower.

2. Add water to cover up vegetables. Cook and simmer on medium until vegetables are tender.
3. Add half of soup mixture into blender. Add bouillon and milk to blender also. Puree several seconds.
4. Add back to saucepan and stir together. Allow to cool and then freeze in smaller containers.
5. Normally potatoes don't freeze well but since you are running the soup through the blender it will work well for the freezer.

CREAM OF CAULIFLOWER SOUP

INGREDIENTS:

- 2 tbsp of olive oil
- 2 onions, chopped
- 3 garlic cloves, minced
- 4 celery ribs, chopped fine
- 2 bay leaves
- 1 -1/2 lbs. potatoes cut in cubes
- 1/2 teaspoon salt
- 1/2 teaspoon pepper
- 15 Cups of vegetable broth
- 2 heads of cauliflower, trimmed and cut into florets
- Heavy cream, milk or evaporated milk

DIRECTIONS:

1. In a soup pan, saute onions, garlic and celery in oil several minutes. Add bay leaves. Add potatoes, salt and pepper.
2. Stir and continue 5 minutes saute all vegetables. Add in broth and cook 15 minutes.
3. Stir in cauliflower and cook an additional 15 minutes until cauliflower and potatoes are tender. Take out bay leaves and blend until smooth.

BROTH BASED SOUP

INGREDIENTS:

- 1/2 tsp cumin

- 1/2 tsp chili powder

- Dash cayenne (optional)

- Dash salt, to taste

- 5 cups vegetable broth

- 1/3 cup couscous, uncooked

- 1/2 cup chickpeas

- 1 tbsp fresh mint, chopped

- 2 tbsp olive oil

- 1 onion, chopped

- 2 cloves garlic, minced

- 1 tsp coriander

- 1 tbsp fresh parsley, chopped (optional)

DIRECTIONS:

1. Saute the onions and garlic in olive oil until soft, about 3 to 5 minutes.
2. Add the spices and cook for one more minute.
3. Add the vegetable broth, chickpeas and couscous. Bring to a slow simmer and cook for 3 to 5 minutes. Stir to fluff the couscous. Allow to sit for a few more minutes, if needed, to allow couscous to finish cooking.
4. Garnish with mint and parsley and serve hot.

Corn Chips in Good Ol' Raw Guacamole

Ingredients:

For the Corn Chips:

- 1/2 tbsp. paprika
- 1/2 tbsp. cayenne
- 3 cups corn
- 1/4 onion

For the Guacamole:

- 1 tomato, diced
- Juice from 1 lime
- 1/2 small pepper, finely diced
- Pinch of Celtic sea salt
- 2 avocados, mashed
- 1 medium purple onion, diced

Directions:

For the Corn Chips:

1. Put all Ingredients: in a food processor and process until the mixture is smooth.
2. Transfer mixture to a Teleflex sheet on a dehydrator tray, making sure that the mixture is evenly spread.
3. Dehydrate for about 12 hours. Flip and then continue dehydrating until it becomes fully dry and crisp.

4. Break the crispy layer according to score lines.

For the Guacamole:

5. In a bowl, combine everything together. Serve the chips with this at the side.

Easy Raw Onion Rings

Ingredients:

For the Almond Milk:

- 4 cups water //
- 1 cup almonds, soaked

For the Onion Rings:

- 1 large sweet onion, sliced
- 1 tbsp. smoked paprika
- 1/2 tsp. ground chipotle
- 1/2 tsp. salt
- 4 cups almond milk
- 1 cup ground flax
- 3/4 cup almond milk pulp

Directions:

1. Prepare the almond milk simply by blending the soaked almonds and the water. Once blended, transfer the mixture to a nutmilk bag and strain. Dehydrate the pulp from the strained milk for 2 hours or until dry.
2. Put the almond milk in a zip lock bag. Soak the onions in milk while the pulp is still dehydrating.
3. Once the pulp is done and dry, put It in a processor along with the flax, spices and salt. It is recommended that you do this in two batches. This way, the mixture doesn't become saturated and too wet for use.
4. Get the onion rings out of the milk and reserve the milk.
5. Cover the onion rings in the flax mixture. Then dip the onion ring slices into milk and then to the flax mixture again.
6. Dehydrate the slices for about 6 hours or until almost dry.

Kale Chips

Ingredients:

- 2 bunches kale, tough spine removed and torn to small pieces
- 3 tbsp. olive oil
- 1 tsp. sea salt

Directions:

1. Wash the kale and spin dry.
2. I a bowl, combine the oil with the salt. Add the kale into the bowl, making sure that everything is well combined.
3. Transfer the mixture into a dehydrator and dehydrate at 115F/46C for about 5 hours or until the kale is crisp.

Lemon-Coconut Squares

Ingredients:

- 1/4 cup coconut oil
- 2 tbsp. coconut nectar
- 1 tsp. lemon rind, grated
- 2 cups coconut, unsweetened and shredded
- 1/4 cup lemon juice, freshly squeezed
- 1 tsp. vanilla extract

Directions:

1. Combine all Ingredients: in a food processor and process until mixture becomes creamy.
2. Line a loaf pan with parchment and then pour the mixture into the pan, making sure that the mixture is spread evenly.
3. Chill for at least one hour and then cut them into squares.

Pepper Poppers, Pine Nut Filling and Eggplant Bacon

Ingredients:

- 10 cayenne peppers, halved and seeds removed

For the Eggplant Bacon:

- 2 tbsp. olive oil
- 2 tbsp. agave
- 1 tsp. smoked paprika
- 1/2 tsp. ground chipotle peppers
- 1 eggplant
- 1/4 cup water

For the Pine Nut Filling:

- 1/2 red pepper
- 2 tbsp. nutritional yeast

- 1 tbsp. smoked paprika
- 1 1/2 cup pine nuts, presoaked for 4 hours
- 1/2 cup cashews, presoaked for 4 hours
- 1/4 cup water
- Juice from 1 1/2 lemons
- Pinch of salt

Directions:

For the Eggplant Bacon:

1. Slice the eggplant into 1/8-inch thick slices using a mandolin and set aside.
2. In a bowl, combine all other Ingredients: and then marinate the eggplant slices in it for at least 3 hours.
3. Dehydrate the eggplant slices at 115F/46C for about 12 hours or until it turns crisp.

For the Pine Nut Filling:

4. Combine all Ingredients: and put in a food processor. Process until the mixture becomes smooth.

Assembling the Dish:

5. Prepare the cayenne peppers. Remember to be careful when cutting and deseeding the peppers and never touch your face while you do this part.
6. Fill the halves with the pine nut.
7. Top each one with the eggplant.

CROCKPOT CORN AND SAUSAGE CHOWDER

INGREDIENTS:

- 1 can (15 oz) creamed corn, undrained
- 1 can (10 oz) cream celery soup
- 1 can whole corn undrained
- 4 cups water
- Corn chowder
- 1 lb breakfast sausage links, cut into bite size pieces, optional
- 3 cups frozen hash brown potatoes or use 3 potatoes peeled and cubed
- Pinch of salt and pepper

DIRECTIONS:

1. Add potatoes, corn and soup to your crock pot. Stir in water and mix until well blended.

2. Season with salt and pepper. If using sausage add to the soup and cook 6 hours on low.
3. While a warm, delicious bowl of vegetable soup can be a healthy addition to any eating plan, a diet that eliminates entire food groups is generally not recommended for sustainable weight loss or wellness.
4. If you enjoy eating soup and would like to benefit from the advantages of plant-based eating, experiment with making healthy soups at home and incorporate them, along with other nutritious meals, into your diet in order to reach and maintain a healthy weight.

MICHAEL ROMANO'S SECRET-INGREDIENT SOUP

INGREDIENTS:

- 1 1/2 teaspoons kosher salt
- 1/4 teaspoon freshly ground black pepper
- 1/4 teaspoon Aleppo pepper or red pepper flakes
- 8 ounces Italian fennel sausage (sweet or hot), casings removed
- 2 tablespoons medium-grind cornmeal (polenta)
- 5 cups Chicken or Vegetable Stock
- 4 cups packed stemmed and coarsely chopped kale or chard leaves, or a combination
- 2 tablespoons olive oil
- 3/4 cup finely chopped onion
- 3/4 cup finely chopped peeled carrot

- 3/4 cup well-washed thinly sliced leeks
- 1 teaspoon finely chopped garlic
- Grated Parmigiano-Reggiano for serving

DIRECTIONS:

1. Heat the oil in a large saucepan over medium heat. Add the onion, carrot, leeks, garlic, salt, black pepper, and Aleppo pepper and cook, stirring, until the onion becomes translucent, 8 to 10 minutes. Add the sausage and cook, breaking it up into small pieces with a wooden spoon, until no longer pink, about 5 minutes.
2. Drain off the excess fat, leaving about 2 tablespoons in the pan. Stir in the cornmeal. Add the stock, stirring, and bring to a boil, then reduce the heat and simmer, covered, for 30 minutes, stirring occasionally.
3. Stir in the greens and cook for 15 minutes more, or until tender.

4. Ladle into bowls and garnish with grated Parmigiano.

TURKEY AND ITALIAN SAUSAGE CHILI

INGREDIENTS:

- 1/2 Jalapeno finely chopped
- 1 dried Bay leaf
- 2 cans Fire Roasted diced tomatoes 14.5 oz each can
- 1 1/2 cups organic Chicken broth
- 1 15.5- ounces can Dark Red Kidney Beans drained
- 1 15.5- ounces can Chili Beans
- 1 tablespoon olive oil
- 1 lb ground Turkey
- 1/2 lb Italian Sausage without casting
- 1 large red Bell Pepper chopped
- Add more salt to taste only if needed

GARNISH:

- 2 cups shredded cheddar cheese or Mexican blend shredded cheese
- 1 cup Sour cream
- Pickled Jalapenos

HOMEMADE CHILI SEASONING FOR 6 SERVINGS

- ½ tsp Onion powder
- ¼ tsp. dried Oregano
- ¼. tsp. dried Parsley
- ¼ tsp freshly ground pepper
- 1 tsp salt
- 1 tsp ground Cumin
- 2 teaspoons Chili powder
- ¼ tsp Cayenne pepper
- ¼ tsp Garlic powder
- 1/2 tbsp. all-purpose Flour /OR Rice Starch

DIRECTIONS:

1. Heat the olive oil over high heat in a large pot and add the ground turkey and Italian sausage. Cook until lightly browned, about 5 minutes, breaking down the meat until it is completely cooked.
2. Add bell pepper, jalapeno, bay leaves and 2 tablespoons of chili seasoning. Stir well and cook for about 2 to 3 minutes at a medium temperature.
3. Add the tomatoes and chicken broth. Bring to a boil, then reduce heat and simmer, for 10 to 12 minutes.
4. Add the drained beans and a whole can of chili beans, then cook, stirring occasionally, for about 10 more minutes. Taste to see if it needs more salt to taste.
5. Serve with cheese, sour cream, and pickled jalapenos if desired.

Double lentil and mushroom barley soup

Ingredients:

- 6 cups vegetable broth or 6 cups water + 1 vegetable bouillon cube
- ¾ cup brown lentils rinsed and sorted
- ½ cup red lentils rinsed and sorted
- ⅓ cup barley rinsed
- 1 teaspoon herbs de Provence
- ¼ teaspoon smoked salt
- Pinch pepper
- 1 teaspoon organic canola oil
- 1 small onion chopped small
- 8 cloves garlic minced
- 14 mushrooms white button or cremini, sliced
- ¼ teaspoon salt or to taste + a pinch more

- 2 cups collard greens chopped & with ribs removed

Directions:

1. Bring a soup pot to a medium heat with oil. Add onions and garlic. Saute until fragrant and the onions are translucent.
2. Add sliced mushrooms to pot along with a pinch of salt. Continue cooking for a few more minutes, stirring occasionally, while the mushrooms release their liquid and soften.
3. Add vegetable broth (or water and bouillon cube, if using), brown and red lentils, barley, herbs de Provence, smoked salt, ¼ teaspoon regular salt, and a pinch of pepper to pot. Bring to a medium high heat, until it has reached a low boil.
4. Turn the heat to low and add chopped collard greens. Stir and cover the pot with a lid. Cook for 25 to 30 minutes, or until the barley is tender.

Smoky corn chowder

Ingredients:

- 1 tablespoon liquid aminos or tamari
- 1 teaspoon liquid smoke
- ¾ teaspoon smoked paprika plus more for garnish
- ½ teaspoon onion powder
- 1½ cups vegetable broth
- 1 cup non-dairy milk unsweetened
- 2 cups baby spinach packed
- 2 tablespoons chiffonade-cut fresh basil plus more for garnish
- ½ teaspoon salt or to taste
- 1 teaspoon sunflower oil or other neutral-flavored oil

- 2 shallots diced
- 1 clove garlic minced
- 4 cups fresh corn kernels or thawed frozen corn
- ¼ cup nutritional yeast
- Freshly ground black pepper to taste

Directions:

1. In a large pot over medium heat, heat the sunflower oil. Add the shallots and garlic to the pot and sauté for 2 to 3 minutes.
2. Add the corn kernels, nutritional yeast, liquid aminos, liquid smoke, smoked paprika, and onion powder to the pot and stir until combined.
3. Add the vegetable broth and nondairy milk to the corn mixture and bring to a boil. Reduce the heat to medium-low and carefully use an

immersion blender to purée about half of the corn kernels (so it remains slightly chunky).
4. Cover the pot, bring the soup to a simmer, and cook for 10 minutes, stirring occasionally. Fold the spinach and basil into the soup and cook for another 5 minutes.
5. Season the soup with salt and pepper to taste and divide it among the bowls. Garnish with a sprinkle of smoked paprika and chiffonade-cut basil and serve immediately.

Creamy vegan tomato soup

Ingredients:

- ½ to 1 teaspoon salt
- Grind black pepper
- 1 Tablespoon nutritional yeast flakes
- 3 Tablespoons tomato paste
- 2 Tablespoons drained oil-packed sun-dried tomatoes + additional oil for drizzling on top
- ¼ to ½ cup non-dairy milk Cashew milk is my favorite
- 1 teaspoon organic canola oil or your preferred neutral-flavored high heat oil
- 1 medium yellow onion chopped
- 1 clove garlic minced
- 1 28-ounce can whole peeled tomatoes including liquid

- ½ cup water
- 1 vegetable bouillon cube
- 1 teaspoon dried oregano
- 1 teaspoon dried basil
- 1 to 2 teaspoons agave syrup optional

Directions:

Bring a soup pot to a medium heat with oil. Add onions & garlic, and saute for several minutes until translucent and fragrant.

Add whole peeled tomatoes with liquid, water, vegetable bouillon cube, dried oregano, dried basil, ½ teaspoon salt, black pepper, nutritional yeast flakes, tomato paste, and drained oil-packed sun-dried tomatoes to pot. Cook for 8 to 10 minutes on a medium heat.

Blend with an immersion blender. Or carefully move soup to a regular blender, blend, and transfer back to the soup pot.

Add ¼ to ½ cup non-dairy milk, depending on your creamy preferences. Taste and add 1 to 2 teaspoons agave syrup if additional sweetness is needed. If more salt is needed, add an additional ½ teaspoon or to taste.

Continue cooking for 5 to 10 minutes longer for flavors to meld and tomato to mellow.

Serve soup in 4 bowls and drizzle with oil from sun-dried tomato jar.

Notes

Masala Tomato Soup

Ingredients:

3 medium sized Tomatoes

1 medium sized Potato

1 tsp green Chili Paste

3 tbsp grated Coconut Pulp

1 tbsp chopped Coriander Leaves

3 tsp Chickpea Flour

1 tsp Jaggery

Salt to taste

¼ tsp Mustard seeds

¼ tsp Asafetida

¼ tsp Turmeric Powder

½ tsp red Chili Powder

1-2 tbsp Cooking Oil (Ghee i.e. clarified butter, Olive Oil, Avocado Oil or Coconut Oil)

Directions:

Finely dice the tomatoes. Then add some water to the tomatoes and cook them well. Once the tomatoes are cooked, make a paste using the blender. (run the paste through a sieve to get an even consistency and to remove the skin grits.)

Boil the potato, peel off its skin and mash it. Then add the mashed potato to the tomato paste/puree crated earlier.

Also add the green chili paste and grated coconut pulp to the patse/puree.

Then add salt, jaggery and chickpea flour to the paste/puree and mix it thoroughly.

Heat the cooking oil in a pan.

Once the oil is hot, add the mustard seeds, asafetida, turmeric powder and red chili powder to the pan.

Once the mustard starts crackling, add the contents of the pan to the tomato paste/puree and mix it well to create the soup mixture.

Then bring this soup mixture to a boil over a medium heat. Garnish with chopped coriander leaves and serve hot.

Tomato Soup in Coconut Milk

Ingredients:

3 medium sized Tomatoes

2 cups of Coconut Milk

1 tsp green Chili Paste

½ tsp Ginger Paste

1 tbsp chopped Coriander Leaves

2 tsp Chickpea Flour

Salt to taste

¼ tsp Asafetida

¼ tsp Cumin Seeds

2-3 Curry Leaves

1-2 tbsp Cooking Oil (Ghee i.e. clarified butter, Olive Oil, Avocado Oil or Coconut Oil)

Directions:

Finely dice the tomatoes. Then add some water to the tomatoes and cook them well. Once the tomatoes are cooked, make a paste using the blender. (run the paste through a sieve to get an even consistency and to remove the skin grits.)

To this tomato puree add the coconut milk, green chili paste and ginger paste. Mix it well.

Then add the Chickpea flour, mix it well and set it aside.

Heat the cooking oil in a pan.

Once the oil is hot, add the cumin seeds, asafetida, and curry leaves to the pan.

Once the cumin starts crackling, add the contents of the pan to the tomato paste/puree and mix it well to create the soup mixture.

Then bring this soup mixture to a boil over a medium heat. Garnish with chopped coriander leaves and serve hot.

Tomato-Onion Soup

Ingredients:

3 medium sized Tomatoes

1 medium sized Onion

1 cup Coconut Milk

1 tsp green Chili Paste

½ tsp Ginger Paste

½ tsp Garlic Paste

1 tbsp chopped Coriander Leaves

1 tbsp roughly grated Almonds (roasted almonds can also be used)

Salt to taste

¼ tsp Asafetida

¼ tsp Cumin Seeds

2-3 Curry Leaves

1-2 tbsp Cooking Oil (Ghee i.e. clarified butter, Olive Oil, Avocado Oil or Coconut Oil)

Directions:

Finely dice the tomatoes and onion. Then add some water to the them and cook them well. Once the tomatoes and onion are cooked, make a paste using the blender. (run the paste through a sieve to get an even consistency and to remove the skin grits.)

To this tomato-onion puree add the coconut milk, green chili paste, garlic paste and ginger paste. Mix it well.

Then add the grated almonds to this soup mixture and bring it to a boil. And then set it aside.

Heat the cooking oil in a pan.

Once the oil is hot, add the cumin seeds, asafetida, and curry leaves to the pan.

Once the cumin starts crackling, add the contents of the pan to the tomato-onion paste/puree and mix it well to create the final soup mixture.

Slightly heat it before serving. (garnish with chopped coriander leaves)

low fodmap tomato soup with meatballs

INGREDIENTS:

FOR THE SOUP

- 1 stalk of spring onion, only the green part

- 6 tomatoes*

- 1 roasted bell pepper (check the ingredients for FODMAPs)*

- 50 g tomato paste

- 500 ml water

- 1 low FODMAP stock cube

- 1 tbsp garlic infused oil

- Oregano and basil

- Pepper and salt

- Optional: fresh basil (as you can see on the picture, I used parsley, but this was only because they didn't have fresh basil in the supermarket anymore and I still had parsley at home)

FOR THE MEATBALLS

- 200 g minced meat (I used half pork, half beef)

- 1–2 tbsp low FODMAP bread crumbs or ground oats (make sure to check the ingredients if you use gluten-free bread crumbs, often high FODMAP ingredients are added)

- ½ tsp paprika powder

- ½ tsp cumin

- Pepper and salt

DIRECTIONS:

- Use a knife to cut a cross into the top of every tomato. Put the tomatoes into a pan with hot water. Like this, the skin will loosen up and you can easily peel the tomatoes. Remove the tomatoes from the water after a few minutes and peel them.

- Cut the tomatoes into pieces and cut the bell pepper into pieces too.

- Heat a tablespoon of oil in a pan.

- Add the green part of the spring onion, the tomatoes, the bell pepper and the tomato paste and fry for a few minutes.

- Add the water and the stock cube. Bring the tomato soup to a boil and leave to simmer for about 20 minutes.

- In the meantime, you can prepare the meatballs.

- Put all ingredients for the meatballs into a bowl. Knead them together well and form little balls with your hands.

- Use a hand blender to make the soup into a smooth mixture. Add salt, pepper, basil and oregano to the soup and taste.

- Add the meatballs to the soup and leave to simmer for another 10-15 minutes. Check if the meatballs are done after about 10 minutes.

- Serve the soup with some fresh basil. You can also add some lactose-free cream if you like.

low fodmap chicken noodle soup

INGREDIENTS:

- 400 g (14.1 oz) chicken thigh fillet

- 2.5 liters (10.5 cups) of stock (use low FODMAP stock cubes)

- 2 medium carrots

- The green part of 6 stalks of spring onions

- 1 red pepper

- 2 tbsp soy sauce*

- 1 tbsp fresh ginger

- 400 g (14.1 oz) mix of oyster mushrooms and mushrooms from a jar (or one of both)

- 150 g (5.3 oz) brown rice noodles

- Optional: 3 boiled eggs, halved

- A slow cooker (I use the Crock Pot Express 6 Quart)

DIRECTIONS:

• Place the chicken thigh fillet in the slow cooker.

• Cut the carrots into slices, the pepper and the spring onions into rings. Save a handful of spring onions for garnish.

• Place the carrot, red pepper, spring onion, ginger, soy sauce and stock in the slow cooker. Stir.

• Set the slow cooker on high for 2 hours and then on slow for another 4 hours.

• Clean the oyster mushrooms and cut into pieces. Rinse the mushrooms from the jar well and let them drain. Set this aside for now.

• After the soup has been cooking for 6 hours, turn off the slowcooker. Pull the chicken meat apart with two forks and return to the pan.

• Taste the stock and season with some salt, pepper or a little extra soy sauce.

- Add the oyster mushrooms/mushrooms to the soup along with the noodles. Put the lid back on the pan and set on low for another 30 minutes.

- Divide the soup over 6 bowls.

- Nice to serve with a boiled egg

low fodmap pumpkin noodle soup

INGREDIENTS:

FOR THE SPICES MIX

- 2 tbsp tandoori spices (make sure no low FODMAP ingredients have been added. The mix that I used contained: paprika, cilantro, salt, cumin, pepper, ginger, chilli, cinnamon and laurel)

- 1/2 tbsp fresh ginger

- 1/2 tsp turmeric

- 1/2 tsp ground cloves

- 1/4 tsp cayenne pepper

- A small handful of fresh cilantro
- A splash of lemon juice
- One stalk of spring onion

FOR THE SOUP

- 200 ml (6.7 oz) coconut milk
- 750 ml (3.2 cups) stock (use a low FODMAP stock cube)
- 400 g (14.1) oz pumpkin in cubes
- 1 tsp fish sauce (leave this out to make the recipe vegan)
- 150 g (5.3 oz) oyster mushrooms
- 1 tbsp brown sugar
- 150 g (5.3 oz) gluten-free noodles
- Fresh basil
- Unsalted peanuts

DIRECTIONS:

- Cut the ginger, cilantro and spring onion into very small pieces. Put those together with all the spices and a splash of lemon juice in a bowl. Make this into a paste using a hand blender.

- Boil the pumpkin cubes in a pan with boiling water for 10 minutes. Drain them well and use a hand mixer to make a pumpkin puree.

- Heat some oil in a soup pan and add the spice paste. Fry this for two minutes while you stir now and then. Add the pumpkin puree, fish sauce and 600 ml stock.

- Scrub the oyster mushrooms clean, cut them into pieces and add them together with the sugar and a pinch of salt to the soup.

- Bring the soup to a boil and leave to boil for about 10 minutes.

- Boil the noodles according to the instruction on the package. Drain them and rinse them with cold water, so they don't stick.

- Add, after 10 minutes of cooking, the rest of the stock and the coconut milk. Leave the soup to boil for another 5 minutes.

- Add some fresh basil and the noodles to the soup and stir together. Turn off the heat and leave the soup to rest for 5 minutes with the lid on the pan.

- Serve the soup with some extra basil and chopped peanuts.

Spinach Cucumber Orange Juice

Ingredients:

- 2 large cucumbers
- 2 oranges peeled and deseeded
- ¼ spoon mix of black salt, mango powder, black pepper, Himalayan rock salt
- 1 fresh bunch of spinach
- 1 fresh bunch of mint leaves

DIRECTIONS:

1. Put the Ingredients: into a juice processor to get juice. Add the spice mix to enhance its taste and drink away.

Spinach Black Carrots Beetroot Juice

Ingredients:

- 2 beetroots peeled
- Juice of 1 lemon
- ¼ spoon mix of black salt, mango powder, black pepper, Himalayan rock salt
- 1 fresh bunch of spinach
- 1 fresh bunch of mint leaves
- 2 large black carrots peeled

DIRECTIONS:

1. Put the spinach and mint first into the juice processor. Follow it with black carrots and beetroots to get healthy iron nutrient juice. Add the spice mix and lemon juice to it and drink instantly.

Carrots Peas Ginger Grape Juice

Ingredients:

- 1 sprig of cilantro leaves
- Juice of 1 lemon
- ¼ spoon mix of black salt, mango powder, black pepper, Himalayan rock salt
- 2 cup fresh peas
- 2 cup grapes
- 2 large carrots peeled
- 1-inch ginger peeled

DIRECTIONS:

1. Source the Ingredients: through the juicer. Pour the juice into glasses. Squeeze juice of 1 lemon and flavor it with the spice mix and relish.

Pineapple Ginger Lemon Juice

Ingredients:

- 2-inch ginger peeled
- 1 cup mint leaves
- ¼ spoon chat masala powder
- 1 pineapple cut in rectangular strips
- Juice of 2 lemons

DIRECTIONS:

1. Put the pineapples, mint leaves and ginger through the juicer. Add lemon juice to it. Pour into glasses. Add the chat masala and savor the taste.

www.ingramcontent.com/pod-product-compliance
Lightning Source LLC
LaVergne TN
LVHW010226070526
838199LV00062B/4738